Restore Health: Disease Reversal

Essays and Book Reviews

JOSEPH E. SCHERGER, MD, MPH

DEDICATIONS

To the many mentor physicians, patients and others who
think that nutrition and lifestyle are the keys to good health
and who wish to use medications sparingly.

CONTENTS

ACKNOWLEDGMENTS

To my assistants Laura Gomez, Janet Riccardi, Jack Hawks and Helen Searing who have aided me in producing this book. I also want to thank Melody Richardson for reviewing the manuscript and making helpful suggestions.

JOSEPH E. SCHERGER, MD, MPH

PREFACE

Restore Health: Disease Reversal

The body wants to be healthy. Evolution has given us multiple mechanisms to repair and restore our body from injuries and illnesses. However, if we repeatedly and continuously damage our body we will overwhelm our repair-and-restore mechanisms and develop a chronic illness.

This book is about restoring health and reversing chronic diseases using healthy nutrition and lifestyle methods. Giving drugs for chronic disease is usually just treating the symptoms or – worst case –simply providing palliative care for chronic diseases. Chronic diseases like Type 2 diabetes or inflammatory bowel disease are not a life sentence. Almost all chronic diseases are reversible! That is not something physicians are trained to do. Physicians are trained to manage chronic diseases, not reverse them.

1

I shifted my medical practice in 2011 to using nutrition and lifestyle methods to reverse chronic diseases. I teach these methods to medical students and residents. I continue to learn from other experts in lifestyle and functional medicine.

Most cancer is caused by nutrition and lifestyle factors, and I have studied cancer remission practices. Seeing patients overcome cancer is very gratifying, and I work with the doctors treating the cancer whenever possible. The methods described here are compatible with the integrative medicine programs at MD Anderson Cancer Center in Houston and Memorial Sloan Kettering Cancer Center in New York.

Premature aging happens to most modern Americans because of nutrition and lifestyle factors. I am medical director of an anti-aging company, Intervene Immune, which provides anti-aging services. An open question today is what we can accomplish by improving our healthspan (the number of years we are healthy) and lifespan using the latest anti-aging techniques.

I have written more than 1,000 medical articles and book reviews. More recently, these have focused on restoring health and reversing chronic diseases. This book is a collection of what I think are the most helpful to restoring health and disease reversal. It is a follow-up to my previous book, *Lean and Fit: A Doctor's Journey to Healthy Nutrition and Greater Wellness*, third edition published in 2019.

I hope you will find much in this book to help you achieve your health goals. I do not claim to have original science or thinking here, but rather have synthesized the work of many others. I am an avid reader of books in lifestyle, functional, and anti-aging medicine. All this material follows solid scientific studies. References are available for all the content.

Joseph E. Scherger, MD, MPH
Indian Wells, California
jscherger@restorehealth.me

PART 1: INTRODUCTION TO RESTORING HEALTH AND DISEASE REVERSAL

Most Chronic Disease is Reversible

Chronic diseases are a recent part of human history. In the past, people went to healers, physicians, or hospitals when they became sick, generally because of infections, injuries, or other maladies. Even cancer was very rare in the past, as described by Mukherjee in *The Emperor of All Maladies* (2010).

The concept of chronic diseases emerged in the 1970s, with high blood pressure (hypertension) being the first. Type 1 diabetes, a complete lack of insulin due to destruction of insulin-making cells in the pancreas, was recognized in the early 20th century. The far more common Type 2 diabetes, due to excess carbohydrates and insulin resistance, emerged with the more recent epidemic of overweight and obesity.

Autoimmune diseases were known in the past, but exploded in frequency in the 1970s, expanding the new medical specialty of rheumatology. High cholesterol became recognized as a disease in the 1980s.

Chronic diseases are often referred to as Western diseases as they are seen in more affluent and industrialized populations. But affluence and industry do not lead to disease; the lifestyle that commonly goes along with them does.

There are six elements to a healthy lifestyle:

1. Nutrition: the most important factor – estimated as the cause of about 80 percent of chronic diseases
2. Physical activity: movement, strength, and balance
3. Stress management
4. Restorative sleep
5. A healthy social life
6. Having meaning and purpose for living

While chronic diseases number in the hundreds, I group them into these categories:

Diseases of carbohydrate overload

The modern American diet and culture are loaded with sugar and refined carbohydrates, which have made the majority of Americans overweight, along with an elevated blood sugar that leads to dementia and many other problems. About 40 percent of Americans are obese, with excess body fat as stored energy. A healthy diet of superfoods such as healthy fats, protein and low carbs can reverse overweight, obesity, prediabetes, Type 2 diabetes, high cholesterol, fatty liver, and metabolic syndrome. Exercise and stress reduction also help this process.

Diseases of inflammation and unhealthy gut microbiome

Inflammatory proteins and fats in common foods may cause systemic inflammation and an unhealthy gut microbiome (dysbiosis), which leads to acid reflux, irritable bowel syndrome and inflammatory bowel disease. Stomach acid is good for us, and the drugs used to reduce stomach acid harm us in the long run. The spectrum of most autoimmune diseases originates in the gut as a result of dysbiosis and small intestinal bacteria overgrowth (SIBO). These conditions can be reversed through healthy nutrition and supplementation.

Diseases of stress

Life today is stressful for most everyone. Achieving a life-controlling stress is an important skill that can be learned, resulting in equanimity during the day and natural restorative sleep at night. Mind and body solutions for stress reduction and optimal mental health are necessary to combat the diseases of stress such as hypertension (high blood pressure), anxiety and depression.

Bones, joints, strength, and balance

Modern lifestyles may give us greater longevity, but our healthy years (healthspan) are in decline. Muscle atrophy and aging of the skeleton leads to many reversible and irreversible problems. Fortunately, the right diet, supplements, physical activity, and technologies such as BioDensity and power plate are effective in naturally restoring strong bones and reversing osteopenia and osteoporosis. Drugs do not do that. Strength training and balance work also can help turn back your physical clock many years.

Chronic fatigue and fibromyalgia

These common health problems respond to optimizing nutrition and lifestyle. With chronic fatigue, improving immune function is vital when a chronic virus is at the core of the problem.

Cognitive decline/dementia

Dale Bredesen (*The End of Alzheimer's*) and Daniel Amen (*Memory Rescue*) have shown that cognitive decline can not only be avoided but even reversed! The three most common causative factors for dementia are elevated blood sugar, inflammation, and toxins. Applying the methods of Bredesen and Amen may preserve cognitive function and even improve cognitive decline.

Cancer remission

While cancer occurs for many different reasons, once it exists it is a metabolic disease. It must be fed and nurtured to cause disease and death. Much has been learned about maximizing your chances for cancer remission and full recovery, with diet and lifestyle leading the way.

Anti-aging

We also have learned much about the biology of aging. We are designed to age and die, and with our modern diet and lifestyle, we accelerate this process. On the other hand, your biologic life can be extended by adopting new practices using diet, lifestyle, and supplementation to delay the processes leading to aging and death.

Chronic disease is reversible, and functional medicine strives to do just that by promoting health rather than treating diseases with drugs and procedures. Using the latest science, practitioners work with clients to reduce or eliminate medications by prescribing nutrition and lifestyle factors. All the elements of a healthy lifestyle are addressed in every person and, whenever possible, real foods are used instead of prescription medications.

Nutritional Healing

Let food be thy medicine and medicine be thy food.
Hippocrates

No disease that can be treated by diet should be treated
with any other means. Maimonides

Tell me what you eat, and I will tell you what you are.
Anthelme Brillat-Savarin

Nutritional healing has a long history in medicine. I had the privilege of visiting the island of Kos in Greece and the location where Hippocrates and his protégés worked circa 500 BCE. The setting was like a spa where nutrition and elements of a healthy lifestyle were taught.

Maimonides was a spiritual healer and a recognized brilliant physician who used food as medicine. Given the central role that nutrition plays in our health it is only natural that what we eat is part of any healing tradition.

Modern Western medicine and medical education favors medications over nutrition for healing. Very little nutrition education is taught in medical school and in continuing education courses. Remarkably, there is no institute for nutrition among the 27 institutes of the National Institutes of Health (NIH).

I studied nutrition while getting a Master of Public Health degree at the University of Washington in 1977-78. I remember that one older professor said that poor people would not get fat because fat calories were too expensive. The rapid development of the fast-food industry in the 1980s proved him wrong.

Like most physicians, I was indoctrinated in the demonization of dietary saturated fat and recommended a low fat, high grain fiber diet for the next 33 years. In 2011, I began reading new concepts in the science of nutrition and realized that much was changing. Since then, I have shifted my medical practice toward nutritional healing, allowing me to prescribe fewer drugs, often getting patients off medications they no longer need, and reversing many chronic diseases.

This book will review important elements of science-based nutritional healing to enable family physicians to prescribe better nutrition for their patients to promote health. I use the term science-based because a deep understanding of human biology and nutrition is more useful than relying solely on randomized controlled trials (RCTs), which are lacking in nutrition science. Moreover, most RCTs are based on a single variable, and nutrition is multivariable by nature.

T. Colin Campbell from Cornell has written about this problem with nutrition research. I found that diving into nutrition science is as exciting as my favorite course in medical school, the pathophysiology of disease. Human biology and the impact of foods are incredibly exciting to learn and, further, to educate patients. The nutrition concepts presented here have been supported by clinical trials.

Carbohydrate Excess and Insulin Resistance

Look around at what has happened to our population. More than 70 percent of Americans are overweight, and more than 40 percent are obese. While obesity has always been with us, this epidemic started in the 1980s when fast food and processed carbohydrates became common foods. The problem is getting worse, and the result is more than weight. Most Americans have metabolic dysfunction and insulin resistance. More than 100 million Americans have prediabetes or Type 2 diabetes.

Our evolutional bodies did not consume large amounts of carbohydrates. Our diets depended on the location where we lived and what food was available; so, diets varied. Carbohydrates consisted of tubers and fruit that was in season. Today, most people consume large amounts of processed carbohydrates, resulting in frequent and greater insulin secretion. Insulin enables our cells to use sugar for energy, a vital function lacking in Type 1 diabetics. Insulin is also a fat storage hormone. David Ludwig at Harvard Medical School and others have shown that the carbohydrate insulin model leading to insulin resistance is the biological basis for overweight and obesity.

Richard J. Johnson, MD, of the University of Colorado has done research showing that storing fat from carbohydrate intake, especially fructose, is a survival reflex and that once fat is stored, our body works hard to keep it or regain it by downregulating our metabolism. What was once used for surviving periods of food scarcity is now leading to an overweight and obese society, given the ready availability of high carbohydrate foods. David Ludwig's research has shown that intermittent fasting periods are the most successful at combatting the lower metabolism of attempted weight loss.

Two important aspects of carbohydrates are the glycemic index and the glycemic load. The glycemic index was developed at the University of Toronto in 1981. A number from zero to one hundred is assigned, based on how high the blood sugar rises after ingestion in a fasting state over 2 hours. The glycemic load is how many grams of carbohydrates a person consumes in a day. Both are important concepts since they are reflected in insulin secretion and fat storage.

Every person has a carbohydrate threshold between 25 and 50 grams daily. The threshold determines whether ingested carbohydrates will be used for energy or stored as fat. Women tend to have a lower carbohydrate threshold than men. Exercise raises a person's carbohydrate threshold on any given day.

David Ludwig has led much of the research on the carbohydrate-insulin model for obesity and its related diseases such as fatty liver and metabolic syndrome. When the body is stressed with repeated high glycemic loads, insulin resistance develops, resulting in elevated blood sugar and increased fat storage. More than 100 million Americans have insulin resistance with Type 2 diabetes or prediabetes.

Robert Lustig at the University of California, San Francisco, has taken the food industry to task for this problem, rather than blame patients or parents. Food advertising is overwhelmingly directed toward sugary sweets and starches. Such foods are addicting, a characteristic not associated with other foods of nature. No one is addicted to walnuts or broccoli, two of the healthiest foods.

It is no coincidence that both Drs. Ludwig and Lustig are pediatric endocrinologists who have seen the children in their clinics become obese, develop fatty liver disease and Type 2 diabetes in large numbers.

These problems can be reversed with low carbohydrate nutrition and intermittent fasting. Obesity is excess fat that is stored energy. The body burns carbohydrates first before it starts burning body fat. If a person stays below his or her carbohydrate threshold on any given day, they will burn fat and lose weight. Go above that threshold and the excess carbohydrates will be stored as fat.

The most effective weight-loss nutrition plans are low carbohydrates with enough fasting time to allow for burning fat, or ketogenesis. This is not a diet, but rather a lifestyle to be followed for the long term. If there is a return to excess carbohydrate intake, the fat will rapidly return.

Women Are Different

Women have greater fluctuations in hormones than men and a standard ketogenic diet often fails in women. Women lose weight slower than men, and given their hormone status, some diet modifications are necessary to achieve greater wellness.

Sara Gottfried, MD, is a Harvard-educated and University of California, San Francisco-trained OB/GYN who was self-admittedly depressed and unhealthy in her 30s. She began to study and write about hormones and women. She is currently a professor in the Department of Integrative Medicine and Nutritional Sciences at Thomas Jefferson University. Her most recent book, *Women, Food and Hormones,* provides a useful guide for treating women to overcome insulin resistance, overweight and obesity.

Nurse practitioner Cynthia Thurlow has had success with helping women lose weight and improve hormonal health through a program of intermittent fasting. She has learned that nutrition practices should vary in the premenopausal, perimenopausal and postmenopausal periods for women.

Inflammatory Foods and Chronic Disease

Twenty-five hundred years ago Hippocrates said, "All disease begins in the gut." A more updated statement would be "all disease begins in the leaky gut" secondary to inflammatory foods. All disease is an obvious overstatement, but the burden of disease caused by foods that trigger leaky gut and dysbiosis is enormous.

We have developed foods in agriculture that were not part of our evolutionary or ancestral diet. Of the three macronutrients, carbohydrates, proteins, and fats, some are inflammatory to the human body. Mostly, these are processed foods or foods that were developed only since the onset of agriculture about 10,000 years ago.

The paleo diet focuses on foods we ate before agriculture and are generally better tolerated. Not all agricultural foods are inflammatory, and every person has a spectrum of foods that may cause inflammation.

Inflammatory foods first manifest in the gut. The gut microbiome is an important organ and consists of 10 times more organisms than we have cells on our body. Eating the ancestral food of nature with variety results in a rich and healthy microbiome. Eating heavily processed foods such as "fast foods" results in an unhealthy microbiome, affecting our mood and gut health. An unhealthy gut microbiome is referred to as dysbiosis.

Leaky gut refers to compounds such as proteins getting through the one cell layer of the intestinal membrane and into the blood stream, thus leading to health problems. Leaky gut happens in the small intestine where colonic bacteria migrate up into the small intestine causing small intestinal bacterial overgrowth (SIBO). Colonic bacteria may even reach the stomach, leading to acid reflux and ulcers.

Stomach acid serves useful purposes such as sterilizing food as part of digestion. Yet with an inflammatory diet, the stomach acid may become excessive and lead to reflux into the lower esophagus, thereby causing tissue inflammation. Severe inflammation of the esophagus is referred to as Barrett's esophagus and may lead to esophageal cancer.

There has been an epidemic increase in acid reflux (GERD) and Barrett's esophagus with the heavily processed standard Western diet. Proton pump inhibitor medications are commonly used to control this, but they are not safe for long-term use.

The most common inflammatory foods are grains, cow's milk, processed vegetable oils and trans fats that come from the hydrogenation of fats in cooking. With patients, I stop or minimize these potentially inflammatory foods first. Some people get inflammatory reactions to the lectin content of legumes, such as tomatoes and beans. The misnomer food allergy is often used for foods that a person does not tolerate. Food tolerances change in a person over time.

Prescribing an anti-inflammatory diet can have major health benefits beyond healing the gut by lessening allergies, skin problems such as acne and rosacea, inflammatory arthritis and other auto-immune disorders, mood disorders and even reversing cognitive decline. Besides the foods mentioned above, high blood sugar also increases inflammation in the body.

The body has systems designed to restore health, and many health problems may be reversed on an anti-inflammatory diet.

Time-Restricted Eating

All tissues in our body have a circadian code that should be understood and respected for good health. Satchin Panda, PhD, at the Salk Institute in San Diego is an expert in this area and has summarized his research in a short book, *The Circadian Code* (2020). In order to allow our tissues time to repair and restore, we should fast at least 12 hours daily without consuming food calories. Water is encouraged for hydration.

I ask my patients to be mindful of when they finish eating every day and avoid any food until at least 12 hours later. I say at least 12 hours because weight loss by burning fat commences in earnest after this 12-hour fast. Each hour of fasting beyond 12 hours provides 50 percent more benefit of fat burning and weight loss. This allows a person to lose body fat with fasting periods of 14-16 hours daily.

Many of my patients are retired seniors who do very well eating two meals a day in an 8-hour period, allowing for 16 hours of fasting with only water, coffee, or tea. Remembering the 12-hour rule allows for flexibility of the fasting time for any given day.

Time-restricted eating, also called intermittent fasting, has many health benefits that have been shown in research. The nutrition formula I use with patients is low carbohydrate, adequate protein, healthy fats, and time-restricted eating. I have found this approach universally effective for weight loss and control.

Healthy Nutrition Options

There is not one healthy diet. Some patients prefer to be vegetarians or vegans, while others follow a Mediterranean, Mexican, or Asian diet just to name a few. The important principle is to eat the real food of nature and avoid heavily processed foods. Among the macronutrients, carbohydrates, proteins, and fat can be unhealthy or healthy. There should be an adequate supply of micronutrients, minerals, and vitamins. If lacking, these can be supplemented. Supplements are not required for a healthy diet with some exceptions such as B12, Vitamin D and minerals for vegetarians and vegans. Vitamin D is an important supplement for seniors who no longer convert Vitamin D from the sun.

My previous book, *Lean and Fit,* and the website, www.leanandfitlife.com, have resources that have been updated here along with recipes and suggested reading.

Reversing Chronic Diseases

Using the principles stated here will allow a person, with their physician, to reverse many common diseases. The formula is to eat the real food of nature that is low in carbohydrates with adequate protein and healthy fats, along with time-restricted eating. This way, patients become ketogenic for part of the day and lose body fat.

Besides overcoming overweight and obesity, Type 2 diabetes, metabolic syndrome, and fatty liver are reversed. Because of the well-being that comes with losing weight and not being frequently hungry, this approach to nutrition is self-reinforcing. One must overcome an addiction to sugar and processed carbohydrates.

In addition, patients should avoid inflammatory foods such as grains, cow's milk proteins, processed vegetable oils and trans fats. Some patients should avoid high lectin food containing legumes such as tomatoes and beans.

On an anti-inflammatory diet, dysbiosis, SIBO and many chronic diseases are prevented or reversed, and other disorders of the GI tract, including gastroesophageal reflux and irritable bowel syndrome. Inflammatory bowel disease such as ulcerative colitis and Crohn's disease may be reversed. Neurodegenerative diseases such as multiple sclerosis and dementia have responded to healthy nutrition.

Becoming a nutritional healer takes study, but many resources are available. The Institute for Functional Medicine (www.ifm.org) and the American College of Lifestyle Medicine (www.lifestylemedicine.org) have courses and certification programs that emphasize nutritional healing. I am rewarded by helping patients become healthier and being a healer. Practicing medicine this way is gratifying and highly satisfying.

The Nature Cure

In Germany, doctors must complete medical school and specialty training before they can become certified in naturopathic medicine. Dr. Andreas Michalsen is Professor of Clinical Complementary Medicine in Berlin at the largest university hospital in Europe. He is board-certified in internal medicine, emergency medicine, nutritional medicine, and physical medicine and rehabilitation. He has published more than 200 articles in leading scientific journals and has collaborated with physicians at Stanford, Harvard, the Mayo Clinic and Dr. Valter Longo at the University of Southern California.

The Nature Cure is a practical guide to the best of natural medicine that is well established in science. The book is a treasure, and endorsed by physicians such as Andrew Weil, Terry Wahls and Wayne Jonas.

The book begins with the basic principles of naturopathy and how it contrasts and complements Western medicine. He calls for collaboration between naturopathic and traditional medical physicians, something that should be encouraged.

In the chapter on therapies of antiquity he makes the case for using leeches for conditions such as osteoarthritis of the knee (amazing results), and for cupping and bloodletting. We should consider these therapies in the U.S. The healing powers of water and fasting are followed with excellent advice.

Dr. Michalsen says that the key to health is using food as medicine. I could not agree more. His nutrition advice is very healthy, and I have only one disagreement. He endorses eating whole grains. He supports Dean Ornish and discusses how unhealthy carbohydrates pushed the surge in obesity.

He follows with the importance of exercise and promotes a "playful" approach to walking. He then goes into mind-body medicine, recommending yoga, meditation, and mindfulness. He reviews "global medicines" such as Ayurveda, Acupuncture and Healing Plants.

Dr. Michalsen then describes how he reverses eight common chronic diseases: hypertension, coronary artery disease (i.e., arteriosclerosis), arthrosis (arthritis), depression and anxiety syndromes, back and neck pain, diabetes, rheumatism, and gastrointestinal diseases. What a great resource this is!

Dr. Michalsen closes the book by giving his strategies for a healthy life and why natural medicine is the future of medicine. Natural Medicine restores health and does not have the exorbitant costs of standard medical practice today. *The Nature Cure* has a prominent place on my bookshelf.

The Pegan Diet

Mark Hyman, MD, is the author of more than 20 books on nutrition. Like me, he trained in family medicine. He is the recognized leader in functional medicine, serving for many years as chairman of the Institute for Functional Medicine and the Cleveland Clinic Center for Functional Medicine. He founded and still practices at The Ultra Wellness Center in western Massachusetts.

Dr. Hyman coined the term Pegan Diet to combine the best of paleo and vegan diets. He began using the term in 2014 after moderating a debate between two founders of paleo and vegan diets and at the end of the debate he was asked what he was. He answered that he must be a Pegan. *The Pegan Diet* is in my opinion the best of Dr. Hyman's books on nutrition and brings together the teachings of his previous works.

These are the highlights of the Pegan Diet:

1. Very low in carbohydrates, especially sugar, flour, and refined carbohydrates of all kinds.
2. Higher in vegetables and fruits, the deeper the colors and the more variety, the better.
3. Higher in good quality fats such as those in olive oil, nuts, seeds, and avocados.
4. Animal products such as eggs and meat should be grass-fed, pasture-raised, and organic whenever possible.
5. Fish should be low in mercury and other toxins.
6. Avoid dairy and grains.

These are the simple rules to live by with your nutrition:

1. Focus on the glycemic load every day and work to stay below your glycemic threshold to lose and maintain a healthy weight.
2. Eat the right fats and stay away from vegetable oils such as canola, sunflower, corn, and soybean. Focus on tree oils such as olive, coconut and avocado.
3. Eat mostly plants. A Pegan Diet consists of 75 percent or more from plants, with vegetables at every meal.
4. Focus on nuts and seeds as a source of protein and healthy fats.
5. Eat beans sparingly, make sure they should be well cooked.
6. Eggs, meat, and fish are more of a condiment rather than the main part of any meal.
7. Fast for 12 or more hours daily to help your body repair and restore, and to burn off excess fat.

The Pegan Diet serves as a "how to guide" with 21 "principles" rather than chapters. The last part of the book describes what to eat for meals, snacks, and desserts. The Pegan Diet is current and comprehensive in that it could be the only nutrition book to recommend. The Pegan Diet is consistent with a healthy Mediterranean diet.

Eat to Beat Depression and Anxiety

Drew Ramsey, MD, a psychiatrist in New York who lives on a family farm in Indiana, introduced me to nutritional psychiatry. I did not realize such psychiatrists existed; it turns out they have international meetings.

Dr. Ramsey's book, *Eat to Beat Depression and Anxiety,* addresses the two most common mental illnesses and how we can eat to avoid and treat them. Ramsey started out in traditional psychiatry, prescribing drugs for mental health conditions. The results were disappointing. He found that healthy foods were much more powerful for healing the brain, and he is now a leading practitioner of nutritional psychiatry.

The emphasis in the book is on what foods to eat, and they are summarized below. Ramsey does not place as much emphasis on what *not* to eat and assumes that people are unwilling to give up their favorite foods. My knowledge and experience suggest that consuming sugar and lots of high glycemic carbs leads to mental health problems. The same may occur with inflammatory foods such as those that trigger gluten sensitivity. To his credit, Ramsey mentions such foods to avoid in the last part of his book.

The best foods to eat to beat depression and anxiety are:

- Leafy greens. Ramsey power player: kale

- Rainbow-colored fruits and vegetables. Power players: red peppers and avocados
- Seafood. Power players: wild salmon, anchovies, and mussels
- Nuts, beans, and seeds. Ramsey power players: pumpkin seeds, cashews, and red beans

(There are healthier seeds such as flax and chia, and healthier nuts, especially walnuts. Red beans can be dangerous if not cooked.)

- Grass-fed or pasture-raised meat. Look for regenerative farms.
- Eggs and dairy. Quality eggs are a brain superfood; eat the yolks. All dairy products should be organic and full fat.
- Dark chocolate. Must be 70 percent or more cocoa, a good source of flavanols, magnesium, zinc, iron, protein, fiber, and potassium.

Dr. Ramsey encourages his patients to transition to these foods gradually to avoid a sudden disruption to the gut microbiome. He emphasizes that a healthy microbiome is critical for brain health since this "organ" has a major impact on our moods. There are more neurotransmitters in the gut than in the brain.

Eat to Beat Depression and Anxiety is a fun read from a very likable psychiatrist and may be helpful in not only encouraging someone to eat healthier, but also getting those affected off medications.

Sleep

Matthew Walker, PhD, is a world expert in the science of sleep. In his book, *Why We Sleep* (2017), he gives us the hard truths about sleep. If we do not get a full night of sleep, we will be impaired, even at the level of a drunk driver. The science says we need 7-9 hours of restful sleep to be healthy. At least one-third of Americans fail to get this amount regularly.

Walker is professor of neuroscience and psychology at UC Berkeley and is the director of the Center for Human Sleep Science. He was previously a professor of psychiatry at Harvard, where they invited him to leave after openly criticizing the university for what they were doing to students during finals week. We all remember the "all-nighters" and how we felt afterwards. Some students die from this.

Unfortunately for physicians, medical training requires repeated sleep deprivation. Nurses and other health care workers may have to work all night and do not get restful sleep of the required length during the day. Our 24-hour society requires this of many other shift workers or people needing to work multiple jobs to support their families. We are a society of sleep deprivation, adding to many health problems, mentally and physically.

All mammals require sleep. As humans, our sleep changes across the life span. From my days of delivering babies, I found it useful to know that newborns will sleep

20 hours in the first two weeks of life, and 16 hours as infants, usually overnight and with two naps. Sleep time daily reduces to 12 hours with one nap as young children. All the way through adolescence 10 hours of sleep is the norm, and school schedules often interfere with this need since adolescents usually do not like to go to bed early. Many junior high and high schools have wisely delayed the start of school to allow students to get an additional 30-60 minutes of sleep.

Trouble sleeping, or insomnia, is one of the most common health problems. Insomnia has many causes and many solutions. Prescription medications for sleep are not a healthy solution and only add to the problems. Sleep hygiene captures the art of good sleeping behavior, and Walker goes into solutions in detail. Our devices, with their blue light interfering with the brain's melatonin release, are just the most recent of the problems. Through evolution, we went to sleep when it became dark, and darkness releases melatonin in our brain. Our indoor world with lighted bedrooms and even television will interfere with sleep.

Sleep is about letting go of what we are dealing with mentally, putting our thoughts and problems away, much like our clothes. The idea of "let me sleep on it" is not to be taken literally in that we are not meant to think about and solve problems when we sleep. Rather, a good night's sleep should refresh us for better decision-making in the morning.

Some of us think that wine or other alcohol may help us sleep. That may be true initiating sleep, but as alcohol wears off, we usually wake up with some arousal interfering with a full night's sleep.

Sleeping through the night without getting up to the bathroom is a luxury not common to middle-aged adults and especially seniors. We should have the skill of going back to sleep with such interruptions.

Meditation such as slow deep breathing helps with this. "Four-square breathing" is becoming popular. This is a slow inhalation through the nose for about four seconds, then hold the breath for about four seconds, and then exhale through the nose for the same amount of time. A brief pause before the next breath completes the four parts of the cycle. Focusing on this type of breathing is an easy form of sleep meditation.

As seniors, our pineal gland, which produces melatonin, becomes calcified. That may be the main reason that many seniors have trouble getting a full night of sleep. Melatonin is not just a sleep hormone, but it has been shown to have antioxidant and anti-aging benefits. It is safe even up to high doses.

My sleep routine is as follows. I initiate sleep at 9:30 or 10 PM and arise 8 hours later at 5:30 or 6 AM. I do this 7 days a week. About two hours before I go to bed, I wear blue light blocking glasses. I can feel my eyes relax. 30-60 minutes before sleep I take a Sleep 3 supplement by Nature's Bounty. This is a time-release tablet that has 10 mg of melatonin along with four herbs and an amino acid known to help with sleep. At the bedside, I have available two 5 mg sublingual melatonin tablets to use as necessary to get back to sleep if I am disturbed or need to go the bathroom. I use four-square breathing to help me get back to sleep. Overall, I am sleeping well and feel rested and productive the next day on this routine. There are lots of options for sleep and everyone should develop a good sleep routine. Walker gives many suggestions in his book.

Being healthy with restorative sleep means that we will spend about one-third of our life asleep. This is not a waste of time, but rather a recipe for a healthy productive life. I encourage you to use this book as a manual for healthy sleeping.

PART 2: DISEASES OF INSULIN RESISTANCE AND METABOLIC DYSFUNCTION DUE TO CARBOHYDRATE EXCESS

Reversing Six Diseases with One Effort

There is one thing a person can do that would reverse six diseases -- reduce the body fat in the trunk. Most Americans have excess body fat in the trunk and that fat is metabolically active causing a host of medical problems. Getting a body composition such as an InBody will specify the problem and provide goals for treatment. These are the six diseases that are directly related to excess body fat in the trunk:

1. Overweight and Obesity. This is the obvious problem of excess body fat.

2. Prediabetes. With 70 percent of Americans being overweight or obese, an elevated blood sugar goes along with that. For the first 30 years of my career, starting in 1971, a fasting blood sugar between 60 and 90 was considered normal. With the overweight and obesity epidemic, most Americans have a fasting blood sugar above 90 so the normal range was changed to 70 to 100. A normal range does not mean a healthy range, it just means what most people have without being labeled as having a disease. We know that a fasting blood sugar below 90 is the healthiest and prevents lots of problems, including cognitive decline. The recognized range for prediabetes is a fasting blood sugar of 100-125.

3. Type 2 diabetes. This disease was first diagnosed around 1890, and by 1971 there were 80 percent of people with diabetes. It occurred almost exclusively in adults and was referred to as adult-onset diabetes. Today, overweight children with excess body fat get this problem, and Type 2 diabetes accounts for 95 percent of all diabetics in America.

4. Fatty Liver Disease. As body fat in the trunk collects, more of it spreads into the liver, thereby causing liver inflammation and damage. This is referred to as non-alcoholic fatty liver disease. Today, in America, more chronic liver disease such as cirrhosis is caused by fatty liver rather than alcoholism or hepatitis.

5. Hyperlipidemia. Body fat in the trunk leads to an unhealthy lipid profile with its increased risk of heart attack and stroke.

6. Hypertension. High blood pressure is the most common chronic disease in America and with every 10 pounds of weight gain, the blood pressure goes up. High blood pressure is a leading cause of heart attacks and strokes. The good news is that with every 10 pounds of weight loss, the blood pressure and risks go down.

All these diseases together are referred to as metabolic syndrome. People with metabolic syndrome become unhealthy and die much earlier.

What is the most effective way to reduce body fat and reverse these diseases? Body fat is stored energy. It only goes away if it is burned. The body is like a hybrid car with two energy sources – sugar and fat. Sugar, which comes from all carbohydrates, is the first-choice ready energy source. A person only becomes a fat burner when the sugar has been burned off. That is why low-carbohydrate diets with intermittent fasting work best. Most Americans consume more carbohydrates than they burn off, and the excess is turned into fat for energy storage. Carbs make a person fat, not eating fats (see Mark Hyman's book *Eat Fat, Get Thin*). Exercise is also helpful in burning off energy and helps a person become a fat burner sooner. Exercise, combined with consuming sugar such as with energy drinks, will not result in fat burning.

Becoming fat in America comes from following the cultural norms of fast food, sweets, and soda. Sugar and carbs are the most profitable food commodities, and they are addictive. Becoming a healthy fat burner means breaking out of these cultural norms, overcoming sugar addictions, and choosing a healthy diet and lifestyle. Best yet, the medical problem list and number of medications is greatly reduced, and a long healthy life is the result.

The Case for a Low Carbohydrate, Healthy Fat Diet

Gary Taubes is a science writer who helped launch the revolution against sugar and away from healthy fats with his 2002 cover article in the New York Times Magazine, titled "What If It's All Been a Big Fat Lie?" He exposed the shoddy science for the low-fat diet recommendations of more than 40 years and how those recommendations resulted in the epidemic of overweight, obesity and Type 2 diabetes.

Best-selling books by Taubes include *The Case Against Sugar* (2017), *Why We Get Fat* (2010) and *Good Calories, Bad Calories* (2007). In his latest book, *The Case for Keto*, Taubes updates the science and provides interviews with nutrition physicians and other health care providers who provide low-carbohydrate, healthy-fat (LCHF) nutrition services in the U.S. and Canada. He also provides his personal experience of being overweight and how he has maintained an LCHF lifestyle for many years.

In a ketogenic eating plan, fat becomes more than 50 percent of your calories. Thus, I emphasize healthy fat since unhealthy fats, as in processed foods, are to be avoided.

Taubes traces the origins of the published history of low-carbohydrate nutrition to two sources: the French physician Jean Anthelme Brillat-Savarin in his 1825 book, *The Physiology of Taste*, in which he concludes that grains and starches are fattening and that sugar makes it worse, and to a London undertaker, William Banting, who reversed his obesity upon the advice of his doctor, and published the bestselling pamphlet, *Letter on Corpulence* (1863). Taubes states that all subsequent articles and books on low-carbohydrate nutrition, including the Adkins diet, are simply reiterations of these works.

David Ludwig has led the academic validation of low-carbohydrate nutrition at Harvard, along with Eric Westman at Duke, Jeff Volek at Ohio State and Steve Phinney at the University of California, Davis. They validate that obesity is an endocrine disorder caused by the fat storage effects of an excess of the hormone insulin induced by carbohydrates. The physics argument of energy-in and energy-out by calories is not valid, yet it persists.

Taubes describes how everyone has a different carbohydrate threshold as to what will cause fat storage. There is no universal daily dietary carb limit (such as 50 grams) that applies to everyone; genetics, a person's metabolism, and whether a person was previously overweight or obese are all important factors for how few carbohydrates a person can ingest without gaining weight. Since we do not need carbohydrates for our health, Taubes recommends abstinence for many people, especially in the weight loss phase of dietary management.

We live in a carbohydrate culture, and the food industry pushes carbs due to their profitability and addictive tendencies. One academic leader of an obesity clinic said he is in the business of treating carbohydrate addiction more than weight management.

I have read three of the four books by Gary Taubes and found each filled with science and practical recommendations. He does not treat patients but expresses how many leading clinicians do so in their centers. Some will find parts of his latest book tedious and repetitious, but overall, it is well worth reading. Taubes summarizes the main points in the introduction for anyone not wanting to get into the details. The final three chapters: Lessons to Eat By, The Plan and Caution with Children, contain valuable information.

Despite the reluctance of many academic departments and weight loss centers (often funded by the food industry), the nutrition debate has been won by the advocates of low carbohydrates as the best and only truly successful long-term approach to weight loss.

Reversing Type 2 Diabetes

In The Diabetes Code (2018), Jason Fung, MD uses "Ockham's razor" to simplify the management of Type 2 diabetes. William of Ockham (1287-1347) was an English Friar and philosopher. He is famous for postulating that with complex problems, the hypothesis with the fewest assumptions is usually correct. Fung is a nephrologist by training and runs the Intensive Dietary Management Program at the University of Toronto.

Fung formulated a new understanding of obesity by developing the argument that obesity is a hormonal illness of excess insulin. With all food consumption, especially carbohydrates, insulin is secreted to drive blood sugar into cells. Insulin is more importantly a fat storage hormone that blocks the burning of fat and causes excess sugar to be turned into fat through lipogenesis. Repeatedly eating carbohydrates causes chronically high insulin levels and the steady accumulation of fat.

Fung stresses the importance of fasting to lower insulin levels enough to begin using body fat for energy. He argues that nutrition for weight loss has been overly focused on what is eaten, and not focused enough on how often we eat. Humans have spent most of their time on Earth eating just one meal a day. Eating three meals a day is cultural and contributes to the epidemic of overweight and obesity, especially with the increased intake of refined carbohydrates.

Fung furthers this same argument to show that Type 2 diabetes is caused by insulin resistance. Doctors have known this for a long time, but Fung simplifies it for a better understanding of how insulin resistance occurs. The repeated secretion of insulin that causes obesity next leads to insulin resistance as a protective mechanism for chronically high insulin levels. This also results in fatty liver early in the disease process.

Insulin resistance further results in the high blood sugar of Type 2 diabetes. Overcome insulin resistance and the blood sugar returns to normal; then Type 2 diabetes is reversed. Fasting is a key part of this disease reversal process.

The approach to preventing and reversing diabetes described in The Diabetes Code is straightforward. The nutrition is healthy fats, low carbohydrates, and intermittent fasting. Healthy nutrition continues for life with good fats: nuts, seeds, fatty fruits, and vegetables such as avocado, quality fish and meat. This is a version of the Mediterranean diet.

All refined carbohydrates and sugars are to be avoided. Further, 12-16 hour fasting periods are built into the daily routine, and adults eat 1-2 meals a day. Water is encouraged to stay well hydrated, and coffee and tea are allowed during fasting periods. Any snacks should be healthy fat and low carbohydrate such as raw nuts. Bone broth or similar foods are used during prolonged fasts to maintain electrolytes.

Obese patients with longstanding insulin resistance often require a prolonged fast to get them started for burning fat, losing weight, and reversing insulin resistance. Fung shows how fat burning does not occur until the insulin levels are low, such as a fasting insulin below 10 mcIU/ml. Fung uses longer fasting periods to get insulin levels low, allowing the body to recover from insulin resistance. To avoid hunger from fluctuating blood sugar levels, the patient is first weaned off refined carbohydrates and started on the healthy fat, low carbohydrate diet.

A minimum initial prolonged fast of 36 hours to three days may be needed to start the process of reversing insulin resistance. For morbidly obese patients, Fung uses initial fasts of seven to 21 days. The longest known medically supervised fast is over one year in a male weighing more than 460 lbs. Micronutrients, ample water and electrolytes are provided during the fast. Coffee and tea are allowed.

Fung describes how many of the drugs used to treat Type 2 diabetes, while they lower the blood sugar, make the underlying disease worse by increasing body fat and increasing insulin resistance. The biggest culprit here is the use of insulin. In the United States, more than 23 billion dollars was spent on drugs for Type 2 diabetes in 2013. In Fung's clinic at the University of Toronto, most patients with Type 2 diabetes have a complete reversal of the disease and are off medications in three to six months.

With *The Diabetes Code*, Fung provides a simple lifestyle approach to preventing and avoiding what has become the most expensive of all chronic diseases. The food industry and the drug industry will not be excited by his method, but it is long overdue for the public to curb the epidemic of obesity and diabetes and the costs of medical care. The methods described by Fung should be taught to medical students and residents and should be used in family medicine offices as part of a lifestyle approach to promoting good health.

Nature Wants Us to Be Fat

We are all survivors of food scarcity. Our ancestors lived through multiple periods of famine. Storing body fat allows us to survive food scarcity. Dr. Richard J. Johnson of the University of Colorado is a leading physician and scientist who studies fat storage as the "survival switch" to protect us from starvation.

Sugar leads to fat storage. The sugar that most leads to fat storage is fructose, a recent discovery. Table sugar is called sucrose, consisting of two sugar molecules in equal amounts, glucose, and fructose. The glucose is used for energy while the fructose goes to the liver to trigger making fat for storage. High fructose corn syrup (HFCS), the most common sweetener used today, is about 65% fructose and 35% glucose. This is why HFCS, used in sodas, salad dressings and many other processed foods, leads to more fat storage and causes the epidemic of fatty liver, overweight and obesity.

Starchy foods like potatoes and rice have a carbohydrate called glycogen, which is chains of glucose molecules and no fructose. These foods are called "safe starches" and do not readily lead to more body fat.

Fruits are high in fructose and are among the most fattening of foods. Bears consume tens of thousands of berries to acquire enough fat to survive a winter of hibernation. Johnson studies many mammals besides humans and describes this biological survival switch among the animal kingdom in this educational book. To control body weight, we should limit fruit to no more than 2-3 servings daily and consume fruits that are less glycemic such as berries, kiwi, and avocados.

Another part of the survival switch is to rapidly accumulate fat once it is lost. A cruel part of having excess body fat is that the body will adjust its metabolism to accumulate fat more than in a person who has been lean.

Losing weight requires burning body fat through low carbohydrate nutrition, especially low fructose. To remain at a healthy weight a person needs to follow a low-carbohydrate nutrition plan as a lifestyle. Periods of fasting or time-restricted eating of more than 12 hours daily also help in burning fat for energy and avoiding a trigger of the survival switch of fat storage.

Nature Wants Us to Be Fat is a great addition to understanding the science behind overweight and obesity. The language is easy enough for anyone to understand. I no longer look at fruit in the same way and am conscious every day to limit my intake.

Time-Restricted Eating May Be the Key to Good Health

When we eat is more important than what we eat. That is the conclusion of Satchin Panda, PhD, leading expert in the field of circadian rhythm research. Dr. Panda is the founder of the Center for Circadian Biology at the Salk Institute and the University of California, San Diego. He has ample research to support his finding. The circadian rhythm is the biological 24-hour clock we all have. In fact, every organ and cell in our body has such a clock that varies according to their function, such as with eating and sleep.

He argues for time-restricted eating (TRE). Our digestive circadian clock needs at least 12 hours daily of not eating to allow for repair and the processing of food to the rest of our body. Breaking this 12-hour code will cause us to gain weight. After 12 hours of fasting, we burn fat and lose weight. This is consistent with the intermittent fasting approach that has become popular since Jason Fung published *The Obesity Code* (2016). Dr. Panda shows that with every hour beyond 12 of TRE the benefits double. Patients will make the most robust changes with TRE in an 8-hour time frame.

After making the case for TRE, Panda recommends other important healthy lifestyle measures such as avoiding processed carbs and other processed foods, exercise, restful sleep, and stress reduction. The section on sleep is especially good in promoting the circadian rhythm for getting 7-8 hours of sleep. I am putting on my red glasses to block out blue light much more regularly since reading the book. I am also reducing my screen time in the evening.

The Circadian Code is a great complement to the other nutrition and lifestyle books I recommend such as those by Mark Hyman, Jason Fung, David Perlmutter, Dale Bredesen and William Davis. I also synthesize this approach of a healthy low carb diet with intermittent fasting in my short book, *Lean and Fit* (2019, Third Edition) and website www.leanandfitlife.com.

PART 3: INTRODUCTION TO DISEASE REVERSAL

The Inflammation Spectrum

Following an anti-inflammatory diet can be confusing. Where do I start? What are the most inflammatory foods? How can I personalize such a diet for the food intolerances I have?

Dr. Will Cole, a functional medicine doctor in Pittsburgh, simplifies this topic in his book, *The Inflammation Spectrum* (Avery, 2019). Dr. Cole points out that lab testing for food allergies and intolerances is usually not specific enough to be helpful. Rather, he uses what I use, an elimination diet plan. Most useful is how his "spectrum" starts with the four food groups that are inflammatory to all or most people. He follows this with four more food groups that show inflammation in some people only. For the second group, these foods may be healthy in some and not tolerated by others. You end up with a personalized anti-inflammatory nutrition plan.

Dr. Cole distinguishes between a food allergy, intolerance, and sensitivity.

A **food allergy** involves the immune system, and there is usually an immediate reaction such as a rash, itching, and hives. In an extreme case there can be anaphylactic shock.

A **food intolerance** is not auto-immune, but rather your digestive system has a reaction reflecting poor digestion, such as gas, bloating or other irritable bowel symptoms. This usually comes from lacking the enzymes to digest the food.

A **food sensitivity** is immune mediated but is a delayed reaction and may be related to how much of the food you consumed. The symptoms are also part of the irritable bowel syndrome.

The first four foods to eliminate are:

1. **Grains** (with or without gluten),

2. **Dairy products** containing lactose and casein,

3. **Sugar and added sweeteners of all types,** and

4. **Inflammatory oils** such as all the processed vegetable oils.

On a healthy diet these are best to be eliminated or avoided. That may be all a person has to do to be on an anti-inflammatory diet.

The second four food groups that are inflammatory to some people are:

5. **Legumes** such as lentils, beans of all types, and anything made from soy. Like Dr. Stephen Gundry, he points to their high lectin content.

6. **Nuts and Seeds**, including almonds, cashews, hazelnuts, and walnuts. I am surprised by this since I list nuts and seeds as "Superfoods" on my website: www.leanandfitlife.com. I must admit that some people tell me they are "allergic" to nuts and seeds.

7. **Eggs**, both whole eggs and egg whites. He comments that many people react to egg whites. I have not seen this since egg whites are mostly the protein albumin. I will start looking for this.

8. **Nightshades**, including tomatoes, peppers, eggplant, white potatoes, and goji berries. These contain alkaloids and are inflammatory to some people. Again, a nod to Dr. Gundry.

Dr. Cole takes the reader through a methodical process of eliminating the foods one at a time by the week and then later reintroducing them one at a time, also by a slow process of a week for each change. This way a person should be secure in the knowledge of what to eat for their most anti-inflammatory diet.

The Inflammation Spectrum is a simple and useful framework for following an anti-inflammatory diet. For more sophisticated coverage of this topic, see Dr. Terry Wahls, *The Wahls Protocol.* (Avery, new edition 2020.)

A Hidden Cause of the Autoimmune Pandemic and How to Get Healthy Again

Hidden chronic infections are common. They are likely a cause of many inflammatory autoimmune diseases and some Alzheimer's diseases. That is the opinion of Steven Phillips, MD, a Yale-trained general internist in Connecticut who became severely ill and recovered from Lyme disease. Dr. Phillips has dedicated his clinical practice to treating a wide variety of under-recognized and hidden infections. Working with one of his patients, singer-songwriter Dana Parish, he has compiled all his knowledge and experience into a new book, *Chronic: The Hidden Cause of the Autoimmune Pandemic and How to Get Healthy Again.*

This book is very scientific, and Phillips' arguments are compelling. After reading this book twice, I began to look at many of my patients differently.

I learned from the AIDS epidemic that some viral infections do not go away. Prior to antibiotics, many bacterial infections such as tuberculosis and leprosy became chronic. Syphilis, if not treated, becomes a serious chronic infection. It is caused by spirochete bacteria similar to that which causes Lyme; if not fully treated, the Lyme bacteria may infect many organ systems. Unfortunately, mainstream medicine, including most infectious disease specialists, do not believe in chronic Lyme disease and other similar infections.

Chronic is loaded with information about what the authors call Lyme Plus infections. These include Bartonella and Babesiosis. There are about 50 types of Lyme bacteria, which makes testing for the disease very difficult. All are spread by insects, especially ticks, and they carry many organisms that can lead to chronic infections.

Diseases shown to be caused by these infections include fibromyalgia, chronic fatigue syndrome, multiple sclerosis, rheumatoid arthritis, lupus, and many others. Terry Wahls, MD (*The Wahls Protocol*, 2014), who suffered from multiple sclerosis, has endorsed this book.

Unfortunately, when most physicians (including rheumatologists) treat these diseases, they use drugs that suppress the immune system, treating only the symptoms while the underlying infection may get much worse. I recently saw a previously healthy woman develop such an illness and die in just two years. Phillips is convinced that our medical model for treating autoimmune diseases is all wrong. They are not actually autoimmune, but rather an immune response to a hidden infection.

Phillips uses the story of Kris Kristofferson to illustrate how these infections can lead to dementia. The famous singer endured cognitive decline, and medicine had nothing much to offer. He was diagnosed and treated for Lyme disease and returned to normal intelligence. How many others out there in memory care centers are experiencing the same?

The recommended treatment of these infections is to strengthen the immune system and use antibiotics on a long-term schedule. In his book *Unlocking Lyme*, William Rawls, MD, shares the success he has had in ridding patients of Lyme disease using herbal therapy about 50 percent of the time. In Phillips' experience, most patients require long-term antibiotics used on a pulsed schedule (such as two weeks on and two weeks off) for six to 18 months. The most common antibiotic used is doxycycline, which is relatively safe for the GI tract and does not disrupt the microbiome or cause C. diff infection. This type of antibiotic is often used in teenagers to treat acne.

Reading this book shook me up. I felt like much of the foundation of my medical knowledge may be wrong. We think we are practicing modern medicine and realize we may still be in the dark ages.

Chronic: The Hidden Cause of the Autoimmune Pandemic and How to Get Healthy Again, has been endorsed by Sanjay Gupta, MD, and notable medical scientists at Harvard, Cornell, and Johns Hopkins University. Give this book to anyone who is chronically unwell, and it may open a corridor for healing if that person can find a physician open to thinking differently.

PART 4: LEAKY GUT-THE KEY TO AUTO-IMMUNE DISEASES

The Microbiome Health Connection

The devastating loss of human life from Covid-19 has highlighted the immense power of tiny, invisible microbes to shape our human experience. Microbes are microscopic organisms, including a variety of widely diverse species such as bacteria and viruses. Bacterial species are highly adaptable to surviving almost any habitat, be it boiling hot geysers, the depths of the darkest ocean vents and even, as we know, in our own human intestines.

"Microbiome" is a term used to describe the vast ecosystem of mostly beneficial microbes that live along the lining of your intestine walls. An explosion of knowledge about the microbiome is ongoing right now as scientists employ genomic sequencing technology to support links between imbalance in the microbiome and just about every chronic disease ranging from acne to Alzheimer's, including diabetes and obesity.

Humans have co-evolved with microbiota in symbiosis over millennia. We rely on friendly gut bacterial species that reside in the large intestine for a myriad of chemical interactions that provide molecules as diverse as Vitamin K to tryptophan. The microbiome helps the human host by digesting dietary fiber in humans who lack the enzymes to digest. In the process of bacterial digestion or fermentation, many beneficial by-products like those mentioned above are released for humans to use. Short-chain fatty acids are especially important byproducts of bacterial fermentation, and their effects have anti-inflammatory actions in the body.

None of this is to say that some microbes are not disruptive and pathogenic. In fact, problematic species often do colonize the gut. The beneficial symbiosis relies on balance—namely the beneficial bacteria outnumbering the problematic, symptom-causing microbes and keeping them in check by outnumbering them.

What can you do to encourage growth of your friendly gut microbiome and discourage the growth of those less than friendly bugs? There are many simple things to start with that, if done well and consistently, can go a long way in supporting your healthy flora.

1. Reduce stress; if your stress level is affecting you negatively, your friendly microbes suffer; be sure to have down time where you allow yourself to relax.

2. Reduce processed foods of all varieties, including "healthy" food that comes in packages.

3. Increase your intake of Dietary Fiber.

4. Reduce caffeine and alcohol intake.

5. Reduce added/refined sugar intake, this includes reducing artificial sweeteners.

6. Minimize the use of acid suppressing medications, (PPIs and H2 blockers,) for example omeprazole or ranitidine.

7. Minimize antibiotic use unless truly necessary.

8. Exercise, dance, swim, practice "Earthing;" spend time outdoors in nature.

Fiber intake is its own special topic and really is the key for many of us who want to optimize our microbiome health and avoid colon cancer, especially those with more conventional American dietary habits. Including specific types of probiotics or prebiotic fiber in our diets can be a targeted approach for certain specific types of problems, but in general most Americans can benefit from simply increasing the diversity of plant fibers in their diet. Prebiotic is the term used to describe fiber sources that help beneficial microbes thrive.

The signature of a healthy gut microbiome is a diversity of beneficial species. This is encouraged by feeding your microbiome a variety of plant fibers and indigestible starches. There are many caveats to fiber intake and many opinions about how certain types of fibrous foods are best consumed or not. A simple starting strategy is to focus on eating a wide variety of plant-based food.

Foods that are rich sources of fiber include all fruits and vegetables, green leafy lettuces and greens, oats, lentils, beans, whole grains, nuts, and seeds. Coconut, chia seed, and flax seed (buy whole seed and grind yourself) are also handy sources of fiber that can be added to many recipes. There are many sources of fiber and indigestible starches that meet even the strictest dietary needs, though it may take a bit of trial and error to find those that work best with your individual physiology. Fiber supplements can be helpful though whole food sources should be prioritized.

There may be minor uncomfortable adjustments to your usual bowel habits as you increase your fiber intake; especially if using supplements. This discomfort should be transitory. Importantly, as you increase your daily intake of fiber be sure to also increase your intake of water or another non-caffeinated unsweetened beverage such as herbal tea.

Whichever dietary path, when you find the best sources of fiber for yourself and your microbiome you should feel better overall. Improved energy, skin tone, digestion, elimination and reduced pain and even improved mood and memory are all possibilities being suggested by microbiome research.

The more comfortable you become with the idea that your microbiome is your partner in health and learn how to support your friendly microbes, the easier it will be to keep your microbiome and yourself in healthy balance.

The Anti-Viral Gut

This is an important book for our times. Integrative gastroenterologist Robynne Chutkan, MD, builds upon her previous books, especially *The Microbiome Solution* (2016), to provide an update for how to have a healthy gut and immune system that will protect us from Covid and other viruses. As much as 70 percent of the immune system is in the gut, so the health of our gut microbiome is crucial to having good health and not succumbing to viral and other infections.

This book is well organized and reads like a course in gut health and immune protection. Chutkan starts with explaining the gut-immune connection. Besides the microbiome and its 100 trillion organisms she uses the term "virome" to describe the 300 trillion viruses on and in the body. Most of these organisms are protecting us.

The second part of the book covers what goes wrong causing dysbiosis, or an unhealthy microbiome. The health of our microbiome depends on what we eat. Highly processed foods cause dysbiosis and leaky gut. An unhealthy gut sets us up for more severe infections, and a large number of other chronic diseases such as autoimmune conditions.

Chutkan then presents an anti-viral gut plan. She covers this comprehensively using the categories of Remove, Replace and Restore. First, you remove medications, practices and foods that are damaging the microbiome. She makes a strong case for keeping your stomach acid and how to get off the acid-blocking drugs that make us vulnerable to infections. Replace involves getting missing or depleted bacteria from food, supplements, and the environment. Specific recommendations are made for foods with some soil and quality probiotic options. Restore includes building up your mucous gut shield layer, which protects you and stops the harm of leaky gut.

These are her key recommendations:

- Eat more plants.
- Choose your carbs carefully (low sugar and eat resistant starches)
- Get ample fiber such as foods high in inulin, such as artichokes, asparagus, garlic, leeks, and onions.
- Eat fermented foods such as sauerkraut, kimchi, and pickles.
- Eat "dirty food" such as from the local farmer's market. Farm yes, factory no.

For the anti-viral gut diet, Chutkan divides foods into green light (eat them abundantly), yellow light (eat sparingly) and red light (avoid entirely). A separate section is devoted to beverages.

After covering other elements of an anti-viral lifestyle such as exercise, sleep and stress management, the book provides lots of recipes to follow.

If everyone followed the anti-viral gut plan our population would be much healthier. We all have a choice of what we eat and how we live. I recommend this book several times every day to patients.

PART 5: DISEASES OF NEURODEGENERATION

The End of Alzheimer's Program

The 2017 book *The End of Alzheimer's* by Dale Bredesen, MD, caused a sensation. For the first time, there was scientific documentation of the reversal of cognitive decline using lifestyle factors. Bredesen, a research professor of neurology at UCLA and founder of the Buck Institute for Research on Aging, first reported on a case of reversal of cognitive decline in 2014. By 2016, he had a small group of successful patients, and by the time his first book was published, he had helped more than 200 patients. Practitioners from all over the world started training in the Bredesen protocol.

The 2017 book highlighted three main causes of Alzheimer's disease: 1) brain atrophy, mainly caused by high blood sugar; 2) inflammation caused by a variety of inflammatory foods and conditions; and 3) toxins due to food contamination and the environment. The treatment program centered on the Mediterranean diet, exercise, quality sleep and stress reduction.

The End of Alzheimer's Program is a more detailed book that many readers requested to better understand the problem and implement lifestyle changes. Bredesen admits he is a researcher and not a clinician. This book updates the research and provides a detailed program with the benefit of two women close to the author.

Julie Gregory has two ApoE4 genes and reversed her cognitive decline using the Bredesen protocol. Julie now spends her time helping others as chief health liaison for Apollo Health, an online health practice. Her description of "A Day in the Life" of living the protocol is outstanding. The second woman is Aida Lasheen Bredesen, MD, Dale Bredesen's wife. She is a trained family physician and integrative health practitioner. Together, these two women present the treatment protocol in great detail.

The recommended diet is called KetoFLEX 12/3 and is ketogenic with intermittent fasting. The Brain Food Pyramid has overnight fasting at the base with non-starchy vegetables and healthy fats next, followed by prebiotics, resistant starch, and probiotics. This program is a refinement of the Mediterranean diet; exercise, restorative sleep and stress reduction are also emphasized as part of the treatment protocol.

Updating the research from the first book, Bredesen has expanded the causes of Alzheimer's disease with a new classification:

Type 1 Alzheimer's is inflammatory or hot. Chronic inflammation is the hallmark of Type 1 and results from the chronic inflammation of insulin resistance with the ingestion of inflammatory foods, chronic stress, and auto-immune conditions.

Type 2 Alzheimer's is atrophic or cold. This type results from inadequate nutrients, hormones or trophic factors needed to support 500 trillion synapses in the brain.

Type 1.5 Alzheimer's is glycotoxic or sweet. Chronic high blood sugar, such as with Type 2 diabetes, causes both brain atrophy and brain inflammation.

Type 3 Alzheimer's is toxic or vile. The results from exposure to toxins such as mercury, toluene, or mycotoxins from chronic mold exposure. Chronic infections such as Lyme and Bartonella fall into this category.

Type 4 Alzheimer's is vascular or pale and results from decreased circulation to the brain due to atherosclerosis. It has been known as vascular dementia.

Type 5 Alzheimer's is traumatic or dazed. This type results from repeated concussions or other head injuries.

The End of Alzheimer's Program provides the detailed treatment recommendations that were lacking in the first book and serves as a manual for treating this increasingly common disease. However, the book is no substitute for training and becoming certified in the Bredesen protocol. Dr. Bredesen acknowledges the contribution of Rancho Mirage physician, Jeralyn Brossfield, MD, to this work.

To look further into Apollo Health, go to: https://www.apollohealthco.com/a-day-in-the-life

The First Survivors of Alzheimer's: How Patients Recovered Life and Hope in Their Own Words

Recovering from Alzheimer's disease is complicated work. Dale Bredesen, MD shocked much of the world with his first book, *The End of Alzheimer's* (2017). The science was clear and published in scientific journals; however, doing the protocol to reverse the disease was not spelled out clearly and was confusing.

His second book, *The End of Alzheimer's Program* (2019), presented the protocol in much more specific detail but was overwhelming for most patients, families and even caregivers. His newest book, written in part by the successful survivors of Alzheimer's disease, is by far the most useful for anyone who is suffering from cognitive decline, as well as for their family and caregivers.

The recovery stories of seven people with well-documented early to moderate Alzheimer's disease are told in detail in their own words. Here are the key takeaways from this book:

- Every person is different. The causes of Alzheimer's disease are varied and multiple. The metaphor is that Alzheimer's disease is like a leaking roof with 36 different holes that must be plugged to stop the damage.
- The nutrition and lifestyle changes are intense and varied from person to person. There is nothing easy about reversing cognitive decline. The person does not have to be perfect every day, but staying on the program is required.
- The treatment program centers around a low-carbohydrate diet of eating only healthy, real foods, with daily fasting of at least 12 hours and three hours before bed. This results in a low blood sugar and low inflammatory markers, required changes to reverse the disease.
- A customized number of brain health supplements are taken by everyone, including what is required for hormone health.
- One hour of exercise is required daily.
- Hormone regulation should be monitored by a physician, and deficiencies in women and men should be corrected with supplements.

- Restorative sleep of six-and-a-half to eight hours daily is maintained, without prescription drugs. Melatonin and magnesium are used to assist relaxing sleep.
- Environmental and dietary toxins are checked for and treated.
- Chronic infections are checked for and treated.
- All causes of stress are reduced or managed in a healthy manner.

A therapist or team of therapists well-educated in the Bredesen protocol (ReCODE) is important to guide a person and family through this process. Not everyone returns to normal cognition, but everyone should benefit from these treatment strategies.

I encourage anyone interested in this topic to read this book and pass it on to anyone suffering from cognitive decline, plus their family and friends. The process of reversing Alzheimer's disease is real if the person works hard enough to achieve optimal health.

The brain, like the rest of the body, wants to be healthy and may return to good health if we stop the insults that cause the problems.

Link Between Parkinson's and Pesticides

Most of us are aware that Alzheimer's disease is on the rise due to high blood sugar and excessive inflammation. These factors are also related to the rise in overweight, obesity and Type 2 diabetes.

Less well known is that the frequency of Parkinson's disease is also on the rise and may be the fasting growing neurological disorder in the world, according to a team of expert doctors and neuroscientists. In their recent book, *Ending Parkinson's Disease: A Prescription for Action* (2020), the authors point to the most common causes of this neurodegenerative condition and what we can do to avoid it.

Alzheimer's and other dementias are due to generalized atrophy and inflammation in the brain. Parkinson's disease reflects the neurodegeneration of specific parts of the brain that use dopamine as the neurotransmitter, the basal ganglia and substantia nigra. Signs of Parkinson's include resting tremors, slow movements (especially in walking), and eventually dementia. Genes and environmental triggers have been suspected, but until now, the main causes have been unknown.

The evidence for agricultural pesticides and herbicides causing the increase in Parkinson's disease is now clear, and these academic neurologists and neuroscientists are calling the alarm. It appears this devastating disease is avoidable.

Agriculture in America is big business, and any health measure that threatens profits is very difficult to enact. This challenge is not new. It took many years to stop the use of DDT in agriculture (still used in developing nations) and asbestos in buildings. Most at risk are the farmers and farm workers regularly exposed to the chemicals cited below, but because there is an approximate 20-year lag between peak exposure and the disease, the cause is not always recognized.

The three major chemicals linked to Parkinson's are paraquat (the most commonly implicated), chlorpyrifos, and trichloroethylene (TCE).

The Environmental Protection Agency (EPA) recognizes paraquat as "highly toxic," but is still used on crops in much of the United States. *Paraquat is banned in 32 countries and listed as a "restricted use" product in California*; however, the authors report that in the past decade, its use throughout our country has doubled.

The nerve toxin chlorpyrifos is the most widely used insecticide in the U.S. The California Farm Bureau Federation reports that in 2013, chlorpyrifos was used to treat almost 60 different crops, including alfalfa, almonds, cotton, grapes, oranges, and walnuts, covering about 1.3 million acres. *Fortunately, in 2020, California banned the sale of chlorpyrifos, and as of December 31,*

2020, agricultural growers are not allowed to possess or use it. However, this doesn't apply to all states.

TCE is used as a solvent to remove grease from metal. It can become toxic by breathing its fumes, ingesting it, or absorbing it through the skin. It is found to cause Parkinson's disease in laboratory animals. *This product has been banned by the EPA for most consumer use, but not entirely for commercial use.*

This book is an important call to action. The Michael J. Fox Foundation has played a leading role in sounding the alarm and supporting action in Congress. We must protect the workers who put food on our table, as well as ourselves and our families, from another human-caused factor causing devastating neurodegenerative disease.

Eating organic produce and carefully cleaning off agricultural residues are especially important today. Pay special attention to the "Dirty Dozen" and "Clean Fifteen" as recognized by the Environmental Working Group and found on its website at <u>www.ewg.org/foodnews</u>

PART 6: CANCER REMISSION

Anticancer Living: Transform Your Life and Health with the Mix of Six

Anticancer Living comes from the husband-and-wife team that led the integrative medicine program at the MD Anderson Cancer Center in Houston, TX. The scientific basis of all their information and recommendations is deep and sound. In many ways, this book is a sequel to *Anticancer: A New Way of Life* by David Servan-Schreiber, MD, PhD (Penguin Books, 2007).

Dr. Servan-Schreiber survived a highly lethal glioblastoma in his brain for 19 years by following an anticancer lifestyle. At the time of his death, Dr. Servan-Schreiber, from the University of Pittsburgh, was teamed with Dr. Cohen for a clinical trial in the methods of anticancer living and their impact on cancer survival and longevity. This trial is ongoing and so far, the results are very promising.

Part One of this book describes the history of what they call the "Anticancer Revolution." Most cancers are much better understood, including the lifestyle insults that lead to the disease. Cancer is about to overtake heart disease as the leading cause of death in the industrialized world. Cancer patients are not helpless and should not simply become passive recipients of cancer treatment. There is much a person can do to improve their chances for cancer remission and for longer survival.

Part Two discusses the "mix of six" interventions in detail. Many personal examples are given. Contrary to the usual method of starting with nutrition, Cohen and Jefferies reverse the order and begin with the psychosocial factors that are so important. First comes a foundation of love and support. Cancer patients who remain well connected to others do much better than those who isolate themselves.

The second intervention is stress management and developing resilience. Every cancer patient is under great stress and managing that is key to better health. Cancer patients usually become stronger in character, and that leads to greater resilience in handling what lies ahead. Controlling stress and developing greater reliance has biological effects that help reduce cancer growth.

Third comes the need for rest and recovery. A diagnosis of cancer is a wakeup call that your life may be out of balance. The body heals during rest so develop a daily schedule that avoids wasting energy and has time for physical and mental restoration.

Fourth comes physical activity. Exercise has tremendous healing powers. Exercise does not have to be vigorous or stressful. Long walks, hikes and swimming are good examples of enjoyable and soothing exercise. Work on preserving and enhancing muscle strength.

Fifth comes food as medicine. Those who follow a plant-based diet have the lowest cancer rates and the greatest chance of remission. Superfoods for cancer are nuts, seeds, and vegetables of a variety of colors. If animal products are consumed, they should be a small part of the diet and the healthiest possible such as grass-fed organic eggs and meat, and wild caught organic fish.

Finally, a low toxic environment is critical to anticancer living. Rid your house of toxic chemicals and limit toxins to and in your body. This chapter is a guide to doing just that.

Appendix materials provide additional guidance for anticancer living. All cancer patients should take responsibility for their optimal health and select an anticancer living life plan. Patients should work with their cancer care providers about treatment, but most do not have a background in the lifestyle factors described here. It is up to you.

Other valuable books to inspire and guide you in reversing cancer and restoring health include:

Anticancer: A New Way of Life. David Servan-Schrieber, MD, PhD. 2017.

Chris Beat Cancer: A Comprehensive Plan for Healing Naturally. Chris Wark 2021.

Radical Remission: Surviving Cancer Against All Odds. Kelly A. Turner, PhD. 2015.

PART 7: ANTI-AGING AND A MAXIMUM HEALTHSPAN

The Forever Dog

This book is much more than about dogs. Dr. Becker is a Functional Medicine veterinarian and with Rodney Habib they are on a mission to save dogs from a life of junk food and poor health practices. Since many people take better care of their dogs than they do themselves, this incredibly eye-opening and informative book will change forever how you feed and treat your dogs, and most likely yourself.

The authors are able to double the life of some of their dogs! Instead of a dog dying of old age around 14 years, their dogs depending on breed can live a happy and healthy life of about 25 years. Yes, 25 years.

As with people, the most important component of a healthy lifestyle is nutrition. The authors take the dog food industry to task and expose the junk carbohydrates most dogs are fed. Most dogs live a life of junk food. Even the healthy and more expensive food brands are full of high glycemic carbohydrates and are lacking in many important nutrients. A few companies dominate many dog food brands, and most trained veterinarians do not know the nutrition their dogs are eating, similar to the lack of nutrition education of most physicians.

The answer is not to just give your dog table scraps. Becker and Habib give you a detailed list of healthy dog foods that you can use, along with sources of healthy readymade meals for those too busy to cook for your dogs.

This bad news-good news book has much more than nutrition information. The authors advise the dog owner to avoid the "triple threat" of stress, isolation, and lack of physical activity. You will learn the difference between a muddy dog and a dirty dog by keeping a dog-friendly environment. Dogs have an incredible sense of smell and nurturing a happy dog is to provide regular "sniffaris," a new word I will remember.

This is a fun book to read or listen to. The knowledge and insights you will take away are huge. The book ends with the section "Pooch Parenting to Build a Forever Dog." There are great quotations, for example: "Whoever said diamonds are a girl's best friend never owned a dog" (Unknown).

Breath: The New Science of a Lost Art

Breathe in, breathe out. Breathe in, breathe out. While breathing is instinctual, breathing *well* is a conscious act. So says science writer James Nestor who, in his illuminating book, *Breath* (2020) compiles some of the science and complexities of breathing. *Breath* is filled with thoughts and techniques, as well as product and service recommendations that can help you become a healthier breather.

Here are a few of Nestor's hallmarks to breathing well:

- **Breathe in through your nose.** Taking breaths in through your nose allows more air to fill your lungs. If you have trouble breathing through the nose, it is important to get that examined. I love standing among oxygen-giving plants and taking a deep breath through the nose.

- **Exhale fully and deeply.** Exhale through your mouth to get the stale air out of your lungs, allowing you to take in more air through your nose.

- **Breathe slowly and less often.** In medicine, a typical breathing rate is 12-16 breaths a minute. That is much too fast and shallow. It is healthy to pause between breaths. Practice taking just four breaths in one minute, spending 15 seconds on each breath cycle. Holding your breath is also a good exercise when followed by deep breathing.

- **Fast breathing** as part of vigorous exercise is also healthy if the breaths are deep and through the nose.

- **Chew to develop the jaw and open the airway.** Unfortunately, modern babies do not chew as much as we did when our species were hunter-gatherers. Our jaws are often undeveloped, which can crowd the wisdom teeth and lead to snoring and obstructive sleep apnea. It is never too late to start chewing more to help develop the jaw and further open your airway for breathing.

In the book, Nestor introduces us to Anders Olsson of Norway, the founder of Conscious Breathing (www.consciousbreathing.com), and his stories are very entertaining. The book also opens our eyes to the history of breathing well as described in this excerpt reiterating a Zhou Dynasty stone inscription from 500 BCE:

In transporting the breath, the inhalation must be full. When it is full, it has a big capacity. When it has a big capacity, it can be extended. When it is extended, it can penetrate downward. When it penetrates downward, it will become calmly settled. When it is calmly settled, it will be strong and firm. When it is strong and firm, it will germinate. When it germinates, it will grow. When it grows, it will retreat upward. When it retreats upward, it will reach the top of the head. The secret power of Providence moves above. The secret power of the Earth moves below.

He who follows this will live. He who acts against this will die.

Young Forever

More than 10 years ago I became interested in two areas of alternative medicine – Functional Medicine and Anti-Aging. Functional Medicine addresses the present health habits of a person in order to prevent or reverse disease. Anti-aging Medicine addresses the future and seeks greater longevity and health span. As I attended conferences in both areas, I was impressed that the anti-aging community tended to look at scientific breakthroughs but did not pay much attention to what people were eating or doing today. Pastries were served during the breaks!

Mark Hyman, MD, is a pioneer of Functional Medicine and besides his own clinical practice at the UltraWellness Center in Massachusetts, he is founder of the Cleveland Clinic Center for Functional Medicine and is board president for clinical affairs for the Institute for Functional Medicine (ifm.org). He has written more than 20 books on nutrition and healthy lifestyle. His latest book, *Young Forever,* bridges Functional Medicine with Anti-Aging, a most welcome development.

In my Restore Health Disease Reversal office I have a shelf of books on anti-aging and *Young Forever* is one of my favorites. It is the most current and comprehensive of these offerings. The book is divided into three parts and 18 chapters. The first part is "How and Why We Age" and looks at both the science of aging and our current nutrition and health habits. Compounds such as Rapamycin, discovered on Easter Island, and Melatonin, not just for sleep, are discussed. There are 10 known hallmarks of aging and Hyman discusses how we can address these with nutrition and supplements. Think clean up the damage to our cells and taking out the garbage.

The second part of the book is "Optimizing Your Health Span and Life Span." Seven core biological systems are described:

1. Nutrients, digestion, and the microbiome
2. Immune and inflammatory systems
3. Energy, keeping our mitochondria healthy
4. Detoxification and elimination
5. Communication systems - hormones, neurotransmitters, and cell-signaling molecules
6. Optimizing circulation and lymphatic flow
7. Structural health and imbalances

The third and final part of the book provides a program for staying "Young Forever." Testing, nutrition including supplements, and lifestyle practices are discussed in detail. The recommendations are comprehensive and practical. This book is a guide to the latest science and health practices to avoid aging as much as possible today.

If everyone followed Dr. Hyman's *Young Forever* program, I suspect life expectancy would increase by 20 years and even more for the number of years we are healthy. I am certainly on board with this.

Lifespan: Why We Age – and Why We Don't Have to

David Sinclair, PhD, is a celebrated aging research professor at Harvard Medical School. He has many videos available on the internet. His groundbreaking 2019 book, *Lifespan: Why We Age-and Why We Don't Have To,* covers the most important three supplements that complement a healthy nutrition and lifestyle. I refer to these as the "Sinclair trio," and they are presented in the Resource section to follow. In brief they are:

- NAD (nicotinamide)
- Resveratrol 100 mg daily
- Metformin (a prescription) 500 mg once or twice daily

NAD cannot be taken orally so it is given in supplements containing NR or NMN, both precursors of NAD.

Most interesting in this book is the story of Sinclair's father who was not well and aging fast upon his retirement in his 60s and is now vibrant in his 80s.

Sinclair argues that aging is a disease, and that disease is treatable. I agree, without a complete denial that aging is inevitable.

CONCLUSION

Removing the insults to our bodies is the key to restoring health and reversing disease. Evolution has given us a multitude of survival mechanisms that will restore our health if we support and enhance these. I hope this book has given you many tools to become healthier and live a longer and richer life.

Use these websites to provide new additional information:

www.leanandfitlife.com

www.restorehealth.me

RESOURCES

Superfoods

There are many lists of "superfoods," known as the healthiest of all foods to eat. Most of these lists overlap with nuts, seeds, many vegetables, avocados, and berries taking center stage. I compiled the following list from several of the authors cited in this book, especially the list of superfoods from Daniel Amen in his books, *Change Your Brain, Change Your Life* (2015) and *Memory Rescue* (2017). I have organized this list into sections for you to choose your foods from. You could eat only the foods listed here and have a nice variety in your diet and achieve optimal health from the nutrition dimension.

I have only included foods that are commonly known and widely available. There are recognized superfoods that are exotic, and some can only be found as supplements. Since these are not necessary for an optimal diet, I have excluded them to avoid excessive costs and keep a superfood diet accessible to everyone.

There are good and healthy foods not listed here and you may eat them for a healthy diet. The most important thing to remember is to strive to eat only the foods of nature in their healthy natural state; organic is preferable. Avoid processed foods whenever you can.

Nuts and Seeds

Tree nuts are the only foods that scientific studies have shown to prevent both cancer and heart disease. Each of the nuts listed here contains different minerals and other nutrients. Having several of these types every week, and eating some nuts every day if you can, is recommended.

Eat these nuts raw and organic if possible. Dry roasting nuts change the health fat into a trans-fat, eliminating much of the healthy nutrition. Also, do not buy these nuts salted to avoid the excessive consumption of salt.

Peanuts are not a nut but a legume and while peanuts have some health benefits, they are not a superfood.

The first three nuts below are the ones I use most commonly in my morning bowl.

Almonds – contain healthy fats, protein, and fiber.

Walnuts – along with healthy fats, including omega-3 fatty acids and fiber, contains Vitamin E, selenium, magnesium, and other antioxidants.

Brazil nuts – these are so high in selenium that only 4-6 nuts should be eaten daily. That is good since they are more expensive than other tree nuts. They also contain zinc, magnesium, thiamine, healthy fat, and fiber.

Pecans – similar to walnuts.

Cashews – a fruit-nut rich in phosphorus, magnesium, zinc, and antioxidants.

Macadamia nuts – high in healthy fats and lower in protein than other nuts listed here.

Seeds rank up with tree nuts as superfoods for a great source of healthy fats including omega-3 fatty acids, fiber, and protein. The following four seeds are widely available and make a great addition to many foods, including your morning bowl. Like tree nuts, the various seeds have different nutrients so look for all of them at different times.

Flaxseed – a layer of these goes into my bowl every morning. Use ground flaxseed since we cannot digest the shell of the seed.

Chia seeds – the energy food of the great long-distance runners of Mexico, the Tarahumara (read *Born to Run* by

Christopher McDougall). Chia seeds are now widely available in the United States.

Hemp seeds – from the hemp plant, rich in protein, healthy fats, fiber, and vitamins. The seeds have no cannabis.

Sesame seeds – despite their simple and pale appearance, these tiny seeds are a rich source of copper, manganese, and other nutrients.

Vegetables

Your daily vegetables should be multi-colored with green being the most important. There are two types of common vegetable superfoods, cruciferous and leafy. There is much overlap between these two categories.

The cruciferous vegetable superfoods include **Broccoli, Brussel sprouts, Cauliflower, Horseradish, Radish,** and **Turnips.**

Broccoli deserves special mention because of its role in DNA methylation, a process of bodily repair, brain health and cancer prevention. Broccoli should be eaten as often as possible. If you do not like broccoli, remember the expression, "There is no such thing as a food you do not like, only foods you do not like yet!" Learn to like what is most healthy.

The green leafy vegetable superfoods include **Arugula, Spinach, Kale, Swiss chard, Watercress, Onions, Cabbage,** and **Collard greens.**

Asparagus does not fit into either of these categories of vegetable, but it is one of the best superfood vegetables.

Legumes are a controversial group of vegetables that are healthy for some and toxic for others. As pointed out by Dr. Steven Gundry in his popular book, *The Plant Paradox* (HarperCollins, 2017), legumes are loaded with lectins used by plants to avoid being eaten. These lectins are inflammatory to some people. These include beans and nightshade vegetables such as tomatoes and eggplant. Be mindful if these vegetables give you acne, rosacea, fatigue, or other symptoms, and avoid them if they do or prepare them as recommended by Dr. Gundry. If they do not bother you, they may be among your superfoods. The Blue Zones all consume legumes, and Dr. John Day, who I follow (www.drjohnday.com), credits legumes as being among the most important foods for healthy longevity.

Fruit

Berries are leading fruits on the superfood list because of their many antioxidants and fiber for our microbiome. **Blueberries, Blackberries, Raspberries** and **Strawberries** are all superfoods. There are other more exotic superfood berries from around the world such as **Acai berries, Goldenberry**, and **Gogi berries**. Have your berries fresh or frozen whenever possible.

Dried berries usually have too much sugar and should be eaten sparingly.

Kiwi and **Pomegranates** are superfood fruits.

Vegetables grow in the ground and fruits grow in trees. Hence, **avocado** is actually a fruit and one of the healthiest foods you can eat because it is filled with healthy fats and protein. Eat one or more avocados every week.

Because most fruits are high in sugar, they are best eaten whole and limited to 2-3 daily. All fruit juice is to be avoided because of the high sugar content. Whole fruits such as oranges, other citrus, peaches, plums, prunes, bananas, and melons are okay to eat but do not rise to the nutrient level of superfoods.

Oils

Olives and **Coconut** are healthy fruits found in different parts of the world and are most known for their healthy oils. **Extra virgin olive oil** is a mainstay of the Mediterranean diet, while **coconut oil** is enjoyed in Asia. These healthy fruits and oils help explain why 3 of the 5 Blue Zones are in the Mediterranean (Ikaria and Sardinia) and in Asia (Okinawa). Cook with coconut oil since it remains stable in the skillet while olive oil breaks down into a trans-fat. **Grapeseed** and **Avocado** also provide superfood oils.

Animal Products

We humans have been omnivores (eating plants and animals) since the beginning of the human species. We should eat mostly plants, and that is why these foods are listed first. The only required nutrient that comes from animals is Vitamin B12, and vegetarians need to supplement that vitamin. The experts I reference in this book all recommend with good science that an optimal diet usually requires some animal-based foods. Vegetarians must work hard to get adequate protein, healthy fats and all the micronutrients only from plants, but it is doable. Also, vegetarians have the lowest rate of cancer and are generally healthier if they focus on nutrition and avoid refined carbohydrates. In my Blogs on www.leanandfitlife.com, I discuss why I do not agree with many of the leading nutrition experts who promote only a whole-food, plant-based diet.

When eating animal products, you have to be very careful to eat only high quality. As Michael Pollan states, with animal foods "you are what you eat." Too much animal feed from farming is based on grains, hormones, and other artificial chemicals, making the product less healthy; they are not superfoods. The foods list below all assume you are buying organically raised foods. Beef should only be grass fed and fish wild caught and low on pollutants.

Dairy

The healthiest part of dairy is the fat. Yes, you read that right. The sugar in dairy, lactose, causes GI upset in most of the world's population. The protein in cow's milk, Casein A, is inflammatory to many people, including infants and children. The saturated fat in dairy has many health benefits, contrary to previous beliefs. Of course, human breast milk is the healthiest form of dairy. Sheep and Goat milk have lactose, but the protein is less inflammatory to humans.

All of this makes **cheese** a superfood! Healthy cheese is not processed, and sheep and goat cheese are the best choices by being the most anti-inflammatory. Cheese has Vitamin K2, which helps direct the calcium in cheese to the bones and not the blood vessels and heart.

European cheeses such as mozzarella, feta, and ricotta are very healthy. The internet has numerous lists of healthy cheeses from credible sources.

I use Half-and-Half in my coffee to limit the plain milk portion. Low fat and nonfat dairy products were a big mistake, resulting from four decades of blaming fat and not sugar for our health problems. Avoid them!

Eggs

Eggs may be eaten every day! David Perlmutter, author of *Grain Brain* and *Brain Maker,* considers eggs as possibly the best food for the brain, which is mostly made of cholesterol. Eggs do not cause heart disease as previously thought. Eggs are not expensive but spend extra to get healthy eggs from an organic supplier with true free-range chickens eating their natural foods.

Fish

Healthy seafood has an advantage over meat since they are not associated with increased cancer rates. Fish from the ocean are healthier than most fresh-water fish except for fresh trout or bass from high altitude. Because our oceans are contaminated with mercury, large fish that eat smaller fish are no longer considered healthy, such as tuna, sea bass, halibut, and swordfish. Dale Bredesen in *The End of Alzheimer's* recommends the SMASH fish. These are:

Salmon

Mackerel (not king mackerel)

Anchovies

Sardines

Herring

Other fish may be healthy depending on location. I also eat shrimp and scallops often.

Meat

There are lots of debates on which meats are healthiest. Some favor poultry such as turkey and chicken, and Daniel Amen favors lamb for its omega-3 content. Grass-fed organic beef and pork may be eaten once or twice a week, and the serving size should be small, 4-6 ounces.

The healthiest meats are organ meats assuming the source is organic and not contaminated with pesticides or other chemicals. Our ancestors thrived on organic meat such as **liver** and **bone marrow.** The Inuit in the far North lived on caribou and got their vitamins and micronutrients mostly from the bones and organ meat, and they fed the muscle meat to their dogs. Dr. Terry Wahls (*The Wahls Protocol)* credits organ meat with helping to reverse her multiple sclerosis.

Bone broth contains many micronutrients and makes an ideal snack or food that may be used during a prolonged fast.

Our body, a product of evolution, has thrived by being omnivores, eating both animal and plant foods. Being only plant or animal-based in your nutrition offers challenges for total wellness but can be done.

Suggested Daily Meal Plan

Healthy nutrition does not require counting calories, even if you want to lose weight. By eating a diet of the real foods of nature, high in healthy fat and adequate protein from healthy sources, the appetite is greatly reduced, resulting in eating fewer calories naturally. Limited carbohydrates, and eating only those in natural foods, does not result in the unstable blood sugar common among those eating grains, sweets and drinking excessive alcohol.

Presented here are what to eat during breakfast, lunch, and dinner. However, as a result of the work of Jason Fung, MD, stressing the importance of intermittent fasting, I recommend that adults eat just one or two meals a day. Here, some choices that I make if I eat during these mealtimes.

Currently, my routine is to eat the breakfast below and then skip lunch, staying well hydrated and alert by sipping coffee with cream. I get two fasting periods each day, about 10 hours between breakfast and dinner and 12 hours overnight. This works well for me with a healthy weight, fasting blood sugar of 85, and a fasting insulin of 4.5. For retired people who have total control over their daily schedule, I recommend the two meals in one 8-hour period, such as between 11 am and 7 pm. That way they get 16 hours of fasting in daily. Remember, this is a usual routine and does not need to be followed every day such as when traveling. The proof of your meal plan is in your results.

Breakfast

My bowl no longer contains cereal, rather:

1. A handful of tree nuts. a combination of almonds, walnuts, pecans, and Brazil nuts.

2. A layer of berries, usually fresh blueberries, but sometimes strawberries, raspberries, or blackberries, or as back-up dried cranberries. About ¼ cup.

3. Three heaping tablespoons of plain yogurt with live cultures, preferably goat milk or coconut milk. Will settle for whole cow's milk if that is all that is available. Alternative or in addition, some plain Kefir.

4. A layer of ground flaxseed, chia seeds or hemp seeds.

5. Unsweetened coconut or almond milk for added moisture. Kefir makes this unnecessary by providing enough moisture. I will use whole cow's milk if that is all that is available.

I may have one or two eggs, hard boiled or fried in coconut oil or butter. Avocado is also an addition to my breakfast if eggs are not available.

After these high protein foods, I may have another fruit such as an orange or banana. The sugar in these fruits is absorbed more slowly after eating protein.

Water, coffee, or tea are the best beverages during the day.

This hearty breakfast will nourish me even with hard work for the rest of the day and make skipping lunch an option for more fasting time.

Lunch

If I have lunch, a salad, preferably with spinach and other vegetables, avocado, nuts, berries and a protein such as shrimp, salmon or chicken breast. No croutons!

Water, coffee, or tea.

Dinner

Have an entrée source of protein such as wild salmon, scallops or other fish. If meat, a modest portion of grass-fed beef such as a petit filet, lamb, pork, chicken, or turkey. I eat fish two times to one over meat.

Combine that with a healthy vegetable such as spinach, asparagus, broccoli, squash or yams, carrots, and tomatoes. Occasionally, I will have whole or Rosemary potatoes. Potatoes are a starch, but they have many nutrients and my exercise is able to compensate for carbohydrates. Sometimes I eat vegetarian and my entrée is tofu or eggplant.

Water and 2-3 ounces of red wine or other alcohol may be used but avoid the grains such as wheat in beer. An ultra-light beer is acceptable, as is white wine.

A modest amount of dark chocolate or fruit may be taken for dessert with the glass of wine. Look for at least 70% cocoa in the dark chocolate.

This meal plan does not require any snacking, and eating between meals is to be avoided. If I skip lunch and want an afternoon snack, I will eat an apple, nuts, or a small piece of dark chocolate. A trail mix of nuts, seeds and modest dried fruit is also a healthy snack if desired. In general, I have learned that I feel better without these things.

Put fasting periods into your day and night schedule. Fasting is very healthy for your metabolism and is much easier when fat and protein are the mainstay of your diet.

Supplements

The Supplements I take

Supplements are just those, things we take to supplement our food choices. They are not a substitute for healthy eating such as the Superfoods

(https://www.leanandfitlife.com/superfoods).

The healthiest and longest living people on earth take little or no supplements. However, there are some important supplements to consider in your journey for greater wellness. Supplements consist of vitamins, minerals, and the micronutrients that our body needs for good health. Some are actual foods like fish oil and herbs. Evolution did not reward us for living beyond our reproductive years. All our body parts and internal chemistry are designed to self-destruct and die. We are all "biohacking" aging to live a long healthy life. These supplements are listed in an order of priority for me as a 70+ senior.

Vitamin D3

The most important supplement for middle aged and older adults is Vitamin D. If Vitamin D were discovered today, it would be called a hormone-like substance. Vitamin D is vital to many body functions, especially our immune system and our bones. It is not present in most foods but is sometimes added to dairy products. When we age, our skin's ability to make Vitamin D from sunlight wanes and many people over age 50 become deficient in Vitamin D even if they are in the sun. This is especially true of seniors over age 65. Hence, Vitamin D is the one vitamin that should be taken by all mature adults. Vitamin D3 is the digestible form of Vitamin D, and I take 5000 IU with 100 mcg of K2 to direct calcium from foods to our bones. This will provide an optimal level of Vitamin D in the blood between 40 and 90 (the normal range of Vitamin D listed in most labs is between 30 and 100).

Magnesium

Seniors do not get as much magnesium from food as younger people and may have muscle cramps or restless legs, especially at night. I take magnesium glycinate 400 mg. every evening for muscle relaxation and sleep.

Melatonin

The pineal gland, which produces melatonin, calcifies with age. Seniors are deficient in melatonin, and this is likely the main cause of poor sleep. I take the time-release product Sleep 3 by Nature's Bounty and have other sleep aids such as 5 mg of sublingual melatonin before 2:30 AM, as needed.

NAD

Nicotinamide adenine dinucleotide (NAD) boosts cellular energy and is essential to all living cells. NAD may slow or even reverse aging and delay the progression of age-related diseases. To get NAD, the supplement is usually NR (Nicotinamide riboside), which converts to NMR (Nicotinamide mononucleotide) to become NAD.

You can buy NMR but is more expensive than NR. I take 300 mg from Life Extension.

Resveratrol

Resveratrol is an antioxidant, anti-inflammatory and immune system moderator that helps protect against a diverse range of chronic diseases and aging. Do not depend on the small amounts in red wine. I take 100 mg daily.

Metformin

Metformin is a time-honored medication for Type 2 diabetes. Diabetic patients taking metformin have a life expectancy even longer than people without diabetes! Research is still exploring this benefit. Metformin reduces the risk of death due to heart disease. It helps with weight loss. Metformin slows some tumor growth and may stop some cancers from developing such as colon polyps. It improves immune function resulting in better outcomes from Covid-19. Diabetics who take metformin have a lower risk of dementia. Metformin is a wonder drug! I take 500 mg every evening.

Harvard anti-aging biologist, David Sinclair, author of *Lifespan: Why We Age and Why We Don't Have To*, considers the trio of NAD, Resveratrol and Metformin together as the best anti-aging supplements.

Turmeric

Turmeric is the spice of curry and has potent anti-inflammatory properties. The active ingredient is curcumin. Curcumin works best when taken in turmeric.

I no longer take ibuprofen or Aleve to avoid the side effects, and turmeric works as well or better. A recent study showed that turmeric is just as effective as omeprazole (Prilosec) for reducing stomach acid. I take 1500 mg daily by Qunol.

Zinc

Zinc has many health benefits and may be the most anti-viral of the supplements to protect against Covid-19, influenza, and the common cold. It is important to know that zinc must be in balance with copper in your body. Copper is an essential micronutrient. 10-25 mg is the dosage range recommended for a viral infection. Zinc lozenges usually have 10 mg of zinc. I take a daily supplement of zinc with copper. I take one of two options: Zinc Balance by Jarrow and Zinc Copper by Solaray.

Glucosamine, chondroitin and MSM.

This combination helps the body maintain strong cartilage, the cushions, or the surface of bones in our joints. I have taken various products of this combination such as Triple Flex by Nature Made.

Nitric Oxide

A Nobel Prize was awarded to the scientists who discovered that taking nitric oxide improved circulation. This led to the development of Viagra and Cialis to help relieve erectile dysfunction. Nitric oxide supplements that are available without a prescription may decrease muscle soreness, lower blood pressure and boost exercise performance. I take the Blood Flow-7 product by

Juvenon. There are many quality nitric oxide products available from reputable sources.

Vitamin B12

Vegans and some seniors close to or over the age of 80 become deficient in Vitamin B12. This can easily be tested for in the blood. If the need is there, take 1 mg or 1000 mcg of Vitamin B12 daily. I get Vitamin B12 in some of my other supplements. B12 shots are not necessary even for people who have pernicious anemia. Contrary to popular belief, Vitamin B12 shots do not give you energy. This **is a** good example of the placebo effect.

Vitamin C

Vitamin C is widely available in fruits and vegetables. Because of its anti-viral benefits, I take a long acting 1000 mg supplement by Nature Made.

Fish Oil

Whether fish oil tables help cardiovascular, or brain health is controversial. I watch the literature go back and forth on this. I take a standard combination of DHA (for brain health) and EPA (for heart health) by Nature Made or another good source like Nordic Naturals. The ratio is usually more EPA than DHA. Some contain another fatty acid ALA (Alpha-lipoic acid) that has antioxidant properties and helps with neuropathy. Neurologist and nutritionist David Perlmutter, MD, considers fish oil and ALA to be vital brain health supplements. Many of the Superfoods like broccoli and spinach are good sources of ALA so I do not consider it a necessary supplement.

CoQ10 or Ubiquinol

Coenzyme Q10, aka Ubiquinol, is an antioxidant that your body produces naturally, and your cells use it for growth and maintenance. Like many other supplements discussed here, levels of CoQ10 decrease as you age. People with heart disease and those taking a statin medication have low levels of CoQ10. CoQ10 is found in meat, fish, and nuts. I also take 100 mg daily by Qunol under the name Ubiquinol, supposedly for better absorption.

SAMe

S-Adenosyl methionine (SAMe) helps the immune system, maintains cell membranes, and helps balance brain chemicals such as serotonin, melatonin, and dopamine. SAMe also contributes to mood elevation. The tablet is light-sensitive, so each one is sealed in foil. SAMe is the one supplement I take first thing in the morning; I take the others after dinner.

Quercetin

Quercetin is a bioflavonoid present in many plants, making it an optional supplement. It has anti-inflammatory properties to complement turmeric. Quercetin also lowers blood pressure, reduces cholesterol, and helps prevent atherosclerosis. I take 500 mg daily from any of the reputable suppliers.

Prostate Health

As a man, I want to do what I can to have a healthy prostate and avoid the common problems, including cancer. Eating the Superfoods and having low body fats help most. Supplementing with saw palmetto is helpful for the prostate. I take the Prostate Health product by Gaia.

DHEA

Dehydroepiandrosterone (DHEA) is a hormone produced in the adrenal glands and is a precursor to making testosterone and estrogens. DHEA peaks at about age 25 and then goes down steadily as you age. It may be helpful for men who are seniors to maintain healthy testosterone levels. I take 50 mg daily.

Spirulina

Spirulina is a food consisting of blue-green algae rich in proteins, minerals, carotenoids, and antioxidants that help protect cells from damage. It may be overkill but as someone who loves Hawaii, I take the tablets from Pure Hawaiian.

JOSEPH E. SCHERGER, MD, MPH

ABOUT THE AUTHOR

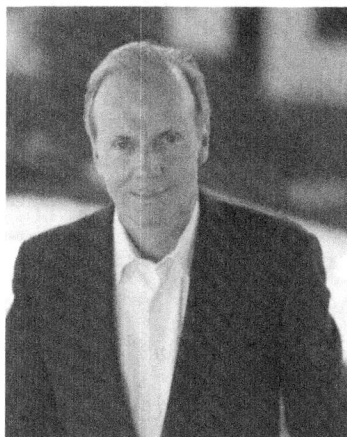

Joseph E. Scherger, M.D., M.P.H., is a family physician in private practice, formerly with Eisenhower Health in Rancho Mirage, CA. He continues his work as a core faculty member in the Eisenhower Family Medicine Residency Program. Dr. Scherger is Clinical Professor of Family Medicine at the Keck School of Medicine at the University of Southern California (USC), University of California, Riverside and the Loma Linda School of Medicine. Dr. Scherger is a leader in transforming office practice and has special interests in nutrition and wellness. He has authored and self-published two books on Amazon, *40 Years in Family Medicine (2014),* and three editions of *Lean & Fit* (2016, 2017 and 2019).

Originally from Delphos, Ohio, Dr. Scherger graduated from the University of Dayton in 1971, summa cum laude. He graduated from the UCLA School of Medicine in 1975 and was elected to Alpha Omega Alpha. He completed a Family Medicine Residency and a Masters in Public Health at the

University of Washington in 1978. From 1978-80, he served in the National Health Service Corps in Dixon, California, as a migrant health physician. From 1981-92, Dr. Scherger divided his time between private practice in Dixon and teaching medical students and residents at UC Davis. From 1988-91, he was a Fellow in the Kellogg National Fellowship Program, focusing on health care reform and quality of life. From 1992-1996, he was Vice President for Family Practice and Primary Care Education at Sharp HealthCare in San Diego. From 1996-2001, he was the Chair of the Department of Family Medicine and the Associate Dean for Primary Care at the University of California, Irvine. From 2001-2003, Dr. Scherger served as the founding dean of the Florida State University College of Medicine.

Dr. Scherger has received numerous awards, including being recognized as a "Top Doc" in San Diego for six consecutive years. He was voted Outstanding Clinical Instructor at the University of California, Davis School of Medicine in 1984, 1989 and 1990. In 1989, he was Family Physician of the Year by the American Academy of Family Physicians and the California Academy of Family Physicians. In 1986, he was President of the Society of Teachers of Family Medicine. In 1992, Dr. Scherger was elected to the Institute of Medicine of the National Academy of Sciences. In 1994, he received the Thomas W. Johnson Award for Family Practice Education from the American Academy of Family Physicians. In 2000, he was selected by the UC Irvine medical students for the AAMC Humanism in Medicine Award. He received the Lynn and Joan Carmichael Recognition Award from the Society of Teachers of Family Medicine in 2012. He served on the

Institute of Medicine Committee on the Quality of Health Care in America from 1998-2001. Dr. Scherger served on the Board of Directors of the American Academy of Family Physicians and the American Board of Family Medicine.

Dr. Scherger serves on the editorial board of *Medical Economics* and has served on numerous other boards. He was a Senior Fellow with the Estes Park Institute focusing on healthy nutrition and wellness. He was the Men's Health expert and a consultant for Revolution Health, 2006-09, and was a physician for eDocAmerica from 2003-2024. He was Editor-in-Chief of *Hippocrates*, published by the Massachusetts Medical Society, from 1999-2001. He was the first Medical Editor of *Family Practice Management.* He has authored more than 600 medical publications and has given over 1,100 invited presentations.

Dr. Scherger enjoys an active family life with his wife Carol, and two sons, Adrian and Gabriel. He has completed 40 marathons, ten 50K and five 50-mile ultramarathon trail runs.

Made in the USA
Las Vegas, NV
08 February 2025